# SOAP Notes Dot Phrase Templates for Medical Records

## By Amanda Symonds

# Table of Contents

# Introduction

If you're working in the medical field, then you know how important it is to have accurate medical records. One way to ensure that your medical records are accurate and up to date is to use medical dot phrases.

Medical dot or smart phrases are a shorthand way of writing medical terms. It  can be used to record medical information quickly and accurately in a patient's medical record. Smart text technology can automatically insert boilerplate sentences into your medical records. For example, when entering "\.dm" for diabetes, the software will create a progress note with all relevant information about this patient including their symptoms and medication regimen which can then be quickly edited accordingly to you and your presenting patient.

Macros, templates, or boilerplate texts can be pre-saved for any medical condition, so you don't have miss vital information during treatment sessions with them! For example, for cardiac patients, medical dot phrases can be used for medical terms such as, "CV" for cardiovascular, "AFib" for atrial fibrillation, and "CAD" for coronary artery disease.

Not only will medical dot phrases help to improve the accuracy of your medical records but can also save you time. When you're recording medical information, using medical dot phrases can help you to record the information more quickly. This can be especially helpful if you're recording medical information in a busy environment and need to maximize the time during consultation with the patients.

Their short, concise nature helps capture only what is necessary about any visit while still being dynamic enough so it can be changed quickly when new clinical information arises in during subsequent follow up with our office or patient.

And finally, medical dot phrases can help to standardize medical terminology across different medical facilities. If you use the same medical dot phrases at different medical facilities, then it will be easier for doctors and other medical professionals to understand your records.

In summary, there are many benefits to using medical dot phrases. First, it helps to ensure accuracy in medical records. Second, it can save time when recording medical information. And third, it can help to standardize medical terminology across different medical facilities.

# SOAP Notes

Types of medical records often used in medical facilities

## 1.  How long should SOAP notes be?

There isn't a definite answer to this answer. The length of a SOAP note will vary depending on the medical facility and the type of medical information being recorded.

## 2.  What is the format of a SOAP note?

SOAP notes are typically formatted with four sections: Subjective, Objective, Assessment and Plan. Listed below are the general contents of each section

·   **Subjective** – information about the patient's symptoms and medical history.

o  Current symptoms and medications described in detail

o  Medical history could be summarised which includes positive and important negative findings

o  Family history of similar illnesses can be included

·   **Objective** – information about the results of physical examinations and tests

o  Physical examination findings should be described in detail

o  Results of any tests performed should be noted with normal average laboratory values and/or vital signs

o  Imaging studied reports should be included

·   **Assessment** – doctor's diagnosis

o  Diagnosis should be based on the information gathered in the subjective and objective sections o  Each differential diagnosis requires indications on which it was based on

·   **Plan** – treatment and management plan for the patient

o  Management plan should be based on doctor's diagnosis. It should include a well detailed clinical care of patient

o  It should also include subsequent follow up plans

o  How the plan was discussed with the patient and caregiver (partner/family member).

o  Whether the patient agrees or refuses the treatment and management plan which include any procedures, medications prescribed or imaging studies during follow up visits

## 3.  What blurb should you include in every SOAP note?

There are a few key pieces of information that should be included in every SOAP note. First, the date and time of the visit should be noted. Second, the patient's medical history should be summarized. And third, the results of physical examinations and tests should be described.

If you're looking for a way to improve accuracy of your medical SOAP records and have an efficient time management routine, then consider using medical dot phrases. It can help to make your SOAP records more accurate and easier to understand. Listed below are some of the examples:

·    Cardiac patients - medical dot phrases can be used for medical terms such as, "CV" for cardiovascular, "AFib" for atrial fibrillation, and "CAD" for coronary artery disease

· Diabetic patients - medical dot phrases can be used for medical terms such

as, "FBS" for fasting blood sugar, "RBS" for random blood sugar, and "HbA1c" for haemoglobin A1c

· Cancer patients - medical dot phrases can be used for medical terms such as, "CA" for cancer, "T" for tumor, and "N" for node

## Dot Phrase Software

StatNote, Epic EMR Smart Phrases and Cerner Auto Text are all popular software programs that use dot or smart phrases in the medical field. We don't promote any particular software in this book.

## Editing Medical Dot Phrase

When you're first creating medical dot phrases, it's important to take the time to edit and customize them. This will help to ensure that they're accurate and that they won't cause any problems during medical audits.

To edit medical dot phrases, you'll need to use the medical record software program. There are many different medical record software programs, and we don't go into them here. In your practice medical record software program, you'll be able to edit and customize the medical dot phrases that you've created.

When you're editing medical dot phrases, there are a few things that you'll need to keep in mind. First, you'll need to make sure that the medical dot phrases are accurate. Second, you'll need to make sure that they're easy to understand. And finally, you'll need to make sure that they won't cause any problems during medical audits.

**Can medical dot phrases cause a problem during an audit?**

Medical dot phrases can sometimes cause problems during medical audits. If you have not taken the time to edit and customize the phrases, then you may find that you are referring to scans or tests that were not taken (and need to be deleted from the medical record).

# Tips about using dot phrases

· Always edit and remove text which does not apply to your patient

· When using medical dot phrases, always make sure to include the medical term in full as well as the abbreviated form. This will help to ensure that your records are accurate and easy to understand

· Re-read your notes to ensure they can be understood by others in your practice and consider how they could be interpreted by someone questioning your patient care in the future

· Always ensure you have read your notes before you sign

# Documenting using dot phrases

**Write a patient letter using dot phrases**

If you're writing a patient letter, you can use medical dot phrases to insert phrases in particular templates and help get the letter produced quickly. Most EMR software already includes templates, but the dot phrases will help you write faster.

## Dictate using medical dot phrases

If you're dictating a medical report, you can use medical dot phrases to abbreviate medical terms. For example, the medical term "EKG" can be abbreviated as "EKG."

This e-book contains dot phrases aimed to improve your experience as a healthcare professional, improving accuracy within medical records and creating an efficient time management routine.

# History of Presenting Illness

| # | Terminology | Dot Phrase | Description |
|---|---|---|---|
| 1 | HPI - Standard | .EDHPI | **age **sex patient with a history of ** is presented to the ED with chief complaint of **. The onset of symptoms was ** days ago. The ** pain is described as ** and currently severe rating at a **/10 with no radiation. Associated symptoms include **. The symptoms are aggravated by ** and have no alleviating factors. Patient denies any **. Patient reported taking ** before arrival for relief of symptoms. No other reported symptoms are mentioned. |
| 2 | | | Patient is **age **sex with a history of ** is presented at the ED with chief complaint of **. The reported pain is at **/10. Associated symptoms include **. The symptoms are not aggravated or have any alleviating factors. The patient denies any **. On arrival ** was noted. No other reported symptoms. Vital signs below. |

3    Patient is a **age **sex who arrives at the ED via ** with chief complaint of **. Patient is accompanied by **. The onset of symptoms began ** and have been ** since day**. Associated symptoms include **. Symptoms alleviated with ** and aggravated with **. Pain is located **, is currently rated a **/10 with ** radiation to **. The patient denies **. No other reported symptoms currently.

4    **age **sex patient with a history of ** has presented to the ED with chief complaint of ***. Symptoms began on **. The pain is rated as a *** out of 10 and described as ***. No other associated signs or symptoms or modifying factors mentioned.

5    The patient is a **age **sex with a history of *** who presents to *** the ED with a chief complaint of ***. Symptoms began *** and have been *** since day **. The patient reports no pain. Associated symptoms include ***. Symptoms are worsened with *** and improved with **. The patient denies ***. Patient denies taking ** for the symptom **.

# Significant Negatives

| # | Terminology | Dot Phrase | Description |
|---|---|---|---|
| 6 | Abdominal Pain | .NEGABDOMINALPAIN | ·nausea ·vomiting ·diarrhoea ·fever ·chills ·flank pain ·dysuria ·hematochezia ·melanotic stools ·chest pain |
| 7 | Back Pain | .NEGBACKPAIN | ·injury sustained to the back ·lower extremity weakness ·bladder or bowel complaints ·paresthesia ·family history of abdominal aortic aneurym |
| 8 | Chest pain | .NEGCHESTPAIN | ·shortness of breath ·palpitations ·nausea ·diaphoresis ·left arm pain ·history of diabetes mellitus ·history of hypertension ·high cholestrol ·history of coagulative disoreds ·family history of heart disease ·leg pain ·leg swelling ·history of DVT or PE |
| 9 | Cough | .NEGCOUGH | ·shortness of breath ·fever ·wheezing ·nasal congestion ·sore throat ·chest pain |
| 10 | Dental pain | .NEGDENTALPAIN | ·recent trauma ·headache ·jaw ache ·neck pain ·fever ·chills ·trismus ·dysphagia ·otalgia ·history of dental pain ·history of dental work |

| 11 | Depression | .NEGGDEPRESSION | ·feeling of sad ·feeling of worthlessness ·feeling of helplessness ·anhedonia ·suicidal ideation ·homicidal ideation ·recent suicidal attempt ·recent self injury ·history of self injury ·alcohol or drug use and abuse ·hyper insomnia |
| 12 | Dizziness | .NEGDIZZINESS | ·localised weakness ·gait instability ·facial droop ·slurred speech ·tremors ·chest pain ·palpitations ·shortness of breath ·syncope ·diplopia ·seizure activity ·nausea ·dysphagia |
| 13 | Extremity Injury | .NEGEXTREMITY | ·excessive bleeding ·trauma sustained to extremities ·back pain ·difficulty ambulating ·gait instability ·localised weakness ·open wounds ·abnormal bone aligment ·paresthesia ·numbness ·cynaosis ·erythema ·other injuries |
| 14 | Fall | .NEGFALL | ·excessive bleeding ·trauma sustained ·loss of consciousness ·head trauma ·hitting head ·back pain·headache ·neckpain ·chest pain ·pain to the extremities |
| 15 | Fever | .NEGFEVER | ·chills ·soar throat ·cough ·congestion ·chest pain ·dyspnea ·headache ·neck stiffness or pain ·skin rash ·altered mental status ·abdominal pain ·back pain ·urinary symptoms |

| 16 | Genito-urinary complaint (F) | .NEG GUFEMALE | ·abnormal vaginal bleeding ·abnormal vaginal discharge ·unusual pelvic pain ·foul smelling discharge ·dysuria ·hematuria ·history of STDs ·itchyness |
| 17 | Groin Pain (M) | .NEG MALE GROINPAIN | ·urinary frequency ·urinary urgency ·dysuria ·hematuria ·testicular swelling ·penile discharge ·history of STDs ·history of inguinal hernia ·back pain ·flank pain ·abdominal pain ·history of diabetes mellitus |
| 18 | Headache | .NEG HEADACHE | ·neck stiffness ·neck pain ·localised weakness ·worst headache ever experienced ·thunderclap headache ·slurred speech ·carbon monoxide poisoning / exposure ·sinus pain / congestion ·trauma sustained ·change in mentation ·paraethesia ·fever ·chills |
| 19 | Motor Vehicle Crash | .NEG MVC | ·excessive bleeding ·trauma sustained ·loss of consciousness ·headache ·neckpain ·back pain ·chest pain ·pain to the extremities |
| 20 | Pediatric Patient | .NEG. PEDS | ·lethargy ·difficulty breastfeeding ·sore throat ·headache ·decreased activity ·fever ·chills ·rash ·emesis ·abdominal pain ·seizure ·urinary symptoms ·history of contact with sick personnel ·sick mother |

| 21 | Seizure | .NEGSEIZURE | ·head injury ·headache ·tremors ·slurred speech ·malaise ·tremors ·localised weakness ·myalgia ·diplopia ·recent sexual history |
|---|---|---|---|
| 22 | Shortness of Breath | .NEGSOB | ·cough ·wheezing ·fevers ·chills ·hemoptysis ·weigh gain ·leg swelling ·chest pain ·palpitations |
| 23 | Sore throat | .NEGSORETHROAT | ·throat swelling ·stridor ·dysphagia ·hoarness of voice ·voice change ·fever ·chills ·rhinorrhea ·congestion ·cough ·nuchal rigidity |
| 24 | Stroke | .NEGSTROKE | ·localised weakness ·facial droop ·slurred speech ·diplopia ·blurred vision ·paraesthesia ·numbness ·pain ·syncope |
| 25 | Syncope | .NEGSYNCOPE | ·headache ·confusion ·lightheadedness ·slurred speech ·seizures ·diplopia ·chest pain ·palpitations ·history of diabetes mellitus |
| 26 | Urinary Complaint | .NEGURINARY | ·dysuria ·hematuria ·flank pain ·abdominal pain ·back pain ·frequency ·history of urinary tract infection ·abnormal penile / vaginal discharge ·fevers ·chills |
| 27 | Vaginal bleeding | .NEGVAGINALBLEEDING | ·current or recent pregnancy ·abnormal vaginal bleeding ·abnormal vaginal discharge ·unusual pelvic pain ·foul smelling discharge ·history of STDs · |

| 28 | Weakness | .NEG WEAKNESS | ·localised weakness ·gait instability ·facial droop ·slurred speech ·tremors ·chest pain ·palpitations ·shortness of breath ·syncope ·diplopia ·seizure activity ·nausea ·dysphagia |

# History of Presenting Illness / Medical Decision-Making Add-ons

| # | Terminology | Dot Phrase | Description |
| --- | --- | --- | --- |
| 29 | Cardiac Risk Factors | .CARDIACRISKFACTORS | ·age ·sex ·overweight ·obese ·BMI ·current everyday smoker ·hypertension ·hyperlipidemia ·diabetes mellitus ·family history of heart disease ·family history diabetes mellitus |
| 30 | Chest Pain Quality Indicator | .CPQUALITYINDICATOR | Quality Indication: Chest Pain Baby Aspirin upon arrival – patient did receive 4 baby aspirin |
| 31 | Heart Score | .TCPHEARTSCORE | Auto-filling populates |

| # | Terminology | Dot Phrase | Description |
| --- | --- | --- | --- |
| 32 | PERC Rule | .PERCULE | The "Pulmonary Embolism Rule-out Criteria" PERC Rule for Pulmonary Embolism<br>[Yes No – 26005] ·   [Yes No] – age greater than or equal to 50<br>·   [Yes No] – heart rate greater than or equal to 100bpm<br>·   [Yes No] – O2 saturation on room air <95%<br>·   [Yes No] – prior history of venous thromboembolism<br>·   [Yes No] – trauma or surgery within 4 weeks<br>·   [Yes No] – haemoptysis<br>·   [Yes No] – exogenous oestrogen<br>·   [Yes No] – unilateral leg swelling à If all variables are negative – PERC Rule can be used to rule out PE. No need for further work-up, as <2% chance of PE.<br>à If any criteria are positive – PERC Rule is not satisfied and cannot be used to rule out PE in this patient |
| 33 | Tetanus | .TETANUS | Tetanus vaccination status {Tetanus Status: Tetanus re-vaccination not indicated} |
| # | Terminology | Dot Phrase | Description |

# Review of Other Systems

| # | Terminology | Dot Phrase | Description |
|---|---|---|---|

| 34 | Review of Other Systems – Symptoms | .EDROS | Systems reviewed and all systems negative except as stated in history of present illness → Cardiovascular symptoms – ·chest pain ·palpitations ·dyspnoea ·pre-syncope ·syncope ·orthopnoea ·peripheral oedema → Respiratory symptoms – ·dyspnoea ·cough ·sputum ·wheeze ·haemoptysis ·pleuritic chest pain → Gastrointestinal symptoms – ·appetite change ·nausea ·vomiting ·dyspepsia ·dysphagia ·weight loss ·abdominal pain ·abdominal distension ·jaundice ·change of bowel habit → Genitourinary symptoms – ·changes in urine output ·changes in urine colour ·infective symptoms ·bladder control symptoms ·obstructive symptoms ·uraemic symptoms → Neurological symptoms – ·visual symptoms ·hheadache ·motor or sensory disturbance ·loss of consciousness ·confusion → Ear, nose, and throat symptoms – ·hearing loss/tinnitus ·otalgia ·facial pain ·persistent nasal discharge ·epistaxis ·dysphonia ·dysphagia ·odynophagia → Musculoskeletal symptoms – ·bone and joint pain ·muscular pain |

# Medical History

| # | Terminology | Dot Phrase | Description |
|---|---|---|---|
| 35 | Active Medical History | .PROBLAMB | Auto-filling populates |
| 36 | Past Medical History | .PMH | Auto-filling populates |
| 37 | Past Surgical History | .PSH | Auto-filling populates |

# Current Medications

| # | Terminology | Dot Phrase | Description |
|---|---|---|---|
| 38 | Current Medications | .EDPTAMEDS | Auto-filling populates |

# Allergies

| # | Terminology | Dot Phrase | Description |
|---|---|---|---|
| 39 | Allergies | .ALLERGY | Auto-filling populates |

# Social History

| # | Terminology | Dot Phrase | Description |
| --- | --- | --- | --- |
| 40 | Pediatric Social History | .PEDSSOCIAL HX | ·does or does not attend daycare ·there is or no passive smoking exposure |
| 41 | Social History | .SOC | Auto-filling populates |

# Family History

| # | Terminology | Dot Phrase | Description |
| --- | --- | --- | --- |
| 41 | Family History | .FAMHX | Auto-filling populates |

# Vitals

| # | Terminology | Dot Phrase | Description |
| --- | --- | --- | --- |
| 42 | General Vitals | .EDVITALS | Auto-filling populates |
| 43 | Orthostatic Vitals | .ORTHOSTATIC | Auto-filling populates |

| # | Terminology | Dot Phrase | Description |
|---|---|---|---|
| 44 | Trauma Vitals | .TRAUMAVITALS | → Time: <br> → Temperature: °C <br> → Pulse: beats per minutes <br> → Respiratory Rate: breathe per minutes <br> → Blood pressure: mmHg <br> → SpO2: |
| 45 | Triage Vitals | .EDTRIAGEVITALS | Auto-filling populates |

# Miscellaneous (Under Vitals)

| # | Terminology | Dot Phrase | Description |
|---|---|---|---|
| 46 | Bladder Scan | .BLADDERSCAN | Auto-filling populates |
| 47 | Visual Acuity | .EDVISUALACUITY | Auto-filling populates |

# Physical Exam

| # | Terminology | Dot Phrase | Description |
|---|---|---|---|
| 48 | Back Pain Neurologic Exam | .EDNEURO | ·5/5 strength in bilateral lower extremities including plantar and dorsi-flexion of extensor hallucis longus ·no foot drop ·normal sensation to light touch ·babinski negative ·2+ patellar and achilles reflexes bilaterally |
| 49 | Knee Exam | .EDKNEE | Left and Right Knee [Positive/Negative/Unknown – 38048]<br>·	[Positive/Negative/Unknown] – varus stress test<br>·	[Positive/Negative/Unknown] – valgus stress test<br>·	[Positive/Negative/Unknown] – anterior drawer test<br>·	[Positive/Negative/Unknown] – posterior drawer test<br>·	[Positive/Negative/Unknown] – patellar apprehension<br>·	[Positive/Negative/Unknown] – patellar ballottement<br>·	[Positive/Negative/Unknown] – McMurray's test |

| 50 | Limited Left Lower Extremity Physical Exam | .EDLLE | Nursing note and vitals reviewed → General: ·alert and oriented X3 ·no acute distress despite patient complaints → Musculoskeletal: · Remining aspects of left lower extremity are unremarkable → Neurological: motor examination reveals +5/5 strength in: · Left hip flexors and extensors · Left knee flexors and extensors · Left extensor hallucis longus ·sensation intact for light touch and skin prick through all dermatomes of the left lower extremities → Vascular: ·left femoral ·left dorsalis pedis ·left posterios tibial pulses are +2/4 → Skin: ·pink ·warm ·dry ·no petechiae ·no purpura ·no ecchymosis |
| 51 | Limited Left Upper Extremity Exam | .EDLUE | Nursing note and vitals reviewed → General: ·alert and oriented X3 ·no acute distress despite patient complaints → Musculoskeletal: · Remining aspects of left upper extremity are unremarkable → Neurological: motor examination reveals +5/5 strength in: · Left triceps · Left biceps · Left brachioradialis · Left intrinsic hand musculature ·sensation intact for light touch and skin prick through all dermatomes of the left upper extremities → Vascular: ·left radial ·left ulnar pulses are +2/4 → Skin: ·pink ·warm ·dry ·no petechiae ·no purpura ·no ecchymosis |

| 52 | Limited Right Lower Extremi ty Physica l Exam | .EDRL E | Nursing note and vitals reviewed → General: ·alert and oriented X3 ·no acute distress despite patient complaints → Musculoskeletal: · Remining aspects of right lower extremity are unremarkable → Neurological: motor examination reveals +5/5 strength in: · Right hip flexors and extensors · Right knee flexors and extensors · Right extensor hallucis longus ·sensation intact for light touch and skin prick through all dermatomes of the right lower extremities → Vascular: ·right femoral ·right dorsalis pedis ·right posterios tibial pulses are +2/4 → Skin: ·pink ·warm ·dry ·no petechiae ·no purpura ·no ecchymosis |
| 53 | Limited Right Upper Extremi ty Exam | .EDRU E | Nursing note and vitals reviewed → General: ·alert and oriented X3 ·no acute distress despite patient complaints → Musculoskeletal: · Remining aspects of right upper extremity are unremarkable → Neurological: motor examination reveals +5/5 strength in: · Right triceps · Right biceps · Right brachioradialis · Right intrinsic hand musculature ·sensation intact for light touch and skin prick through all dermatomes of the left upper extremities → Vascular: ·right radial ·right ulnar pulses are +2/4 → Skin: ·pink ·warm ·dry ·no petechiae ·no purpura ·no ecchymosis |

| 54 | Lower Extremity Strength Exam | .LESTRENGTH | Strength 5/5 in: · Hip flexors and extensors<br>· Quadriceps<br>· Hamstrings<br>· Gastrocnemius<br>· Extensor hallucis longus<br>· Tibialis anterior |
|---|---|---|---|

| 55 | Pediatric (4 years or less) Physical Exam | .EDPEDS | Nursing note and vitals reviewed → General: ·alert and oriented X3 ·no acute distressd despite patient complaints ·appropriately interactive
→    HEENT: ·        Head – ·normocephalic ·atraumatic
·        Eyes – ·pupils equal 3mm in size, round and reactive
·        Ears – ·otorrhea ·heamotympanum ·pearly grey tympanic membrane
·        Nose – ·epitaxis ·septal hematoma ·nares patent bilaterally
·        Throat – ·oropharynx clear ·pink ·moist ·active bleeding or intraoral injuries ·no pharyngeal erythema or exudate →    Neck: ·supple ·trachea midline ·no lymphadenopathy ·no masses
→    Chest: ·symmetrical chest movement ·no subcutaneous emphysema ·lungs are clear on auscultations bilaterally ·no crepitus ·no rhochi ·no rales
→    Cardiovascular: ·regular rate and rhythm of pulse ·normal S1 S2 sounds ·no murmurs ·no rubs ·no gallops ·no muffled heart tones
→    Vascular: +2/4 bilaterally equal – ·radial ·femoral ·dorsalis pedis arteries·capillaries refill  more than two seconds
→    Abdomen: ·soft ·non distended (localled or generalised) ·non tender (no guarding, no rebound tenderness) ·active bowel sounds in all 4 quadrants ·no |

| 56 | Pediatric (less than 2 years) Physical Exam | .PEDIATRICPHYSICAL | Nursing note and vitals reviewed → HEENT: · Head – ·normocephalic ·atraumatic<br>· Eyes – ·pupils equal, round and reactive, ·sclera are white<br>· Ears – ·no otorrhea ·no heamotympanum ·clear tympanic membrane<br>· Nose – ·no epitaxis ·septal hematoma ·nares patent bilaterally ·no rhinorrhea<br>· Throat – ·oropharynx clear ·pink ·moist and no exudate ·no active bleeding or intraoral injuries ·no asymmetry of posterior phraynx →<br>Neck: ·supple ·trachea midline ·no Jugular Venous Distension ·no carotid bruits ·no lymphadenopathy ·no midline C spine tenderness and no midline tenderness on palpation<br>→ Chest: ·symmetrical chest movement ·no crepitus ·no retraction<br>→ Lungs: ·lungs are clear on auscultations bilaterally ·no crepitus ·no rhochi ·no rales<br>→ Back: ·no evidence trauma sustained<br>→ Cardiovascular: ·regular ·no murmurs ·no rubs ·no gallops·no muffled heart tones<br>→ Vascular: +2/4 bilaterally equal – ·radial ·femoral ·dorsalis pedis arteries<br>→ Abdomen: ·soft and non tender (no guarding, no rebound tenderness) ·active bowel sounds in all 4 quadrants ·no palpable mass |

| 57 | Physical Exam | .EDPE X | Nursing note and vitals reviewed → |
|---|---|---|---|

General: ·alert and oriented X3 ·no significant distress despite patient complaints

→ HEENT: · Head – ·normocephalic ·atraumatic

· Eyes – ·pupils equal 3mm in size, round and reactive

· Ears – ·otorrhea ·heamotympanum ·pearly grey tympanic membrane

· Nose – ·epitaxis ·septal hematoma ·nares patent bilaterally

· Throat – ·oropharynx clear ·pink ·moist ·active bleeding or intraoral injuries

→ Neck: ·trachea midline ·no Jugular Venous Distension ·no carotid bruits ·no lymphadenopathy ·no midline C spine tenderness

→ Chest: ·symmetrical chest movement ·non-tender chest wall ·no subcutaneous emphysema ·lungs are clear on auscultations bilaterally ·no crepitus ·no rhochi ·no rales

→ Cardiovascular: ·regular rate and rhythm of pulse ·normal S1 S2 sounds ·no murmurs ·no rubs ·no gallops ·no muffled heart tones

→ Vascular: +2/4 bilaterally equal – ·radial ·femoral ·dorsalis pedis arteries

→ Abdomen: ·soft ·non distended (localled or generalised) ·non tender (no guarding, no rebound tenderness) ·active bowel sounds in all 4 quadrants ·no selt belt sign

→ Pelvis: stable to rock ·no

| 58 | Physical Exam | .EDPE X | Nursing note and vitals reviewed → General: ·patient lying on cart ·alert ·no significant distress<br>→ HEENT: · Head – ·normocephalic ·atraumatic<br>· Eyes – ·pupils equal, round and reactive<br>· Ears – ·no otorrhea ·no heamotympanum ·clear tympanic membrane<br>· Nose – ·epitaxis ·septal hematoma ·nares patent bilaterally ·no rhinorrhea<br>· Throat – ·oropharynx clear ·pink ·moist ·active bleeding or intraoral injuries<br>→ Neck: ·supple ·trachea midline ·no Jugular Venous Distension ·no carotid bruits ·no lymphadenopathy ·no midline C spine tenderness and no midline tenderness on palpation<br>→ Chest: ·symmetrical chest movement ·no subcutaneous emphysema<br>→ Lungs: ·lungs are clear on auscultations bilaterally ·no crepitus ·no rhochi ·no rales<br>→ Back: ·no midline or paraspinal tenderness on palpation ·no trauma sustained ·no CVA tenderness ·no erythema ·no increased calor<br>→ Cardiovascular: ·normal S1 S2 sounds ·no murmurs ·no rubs ·no gallops·no muffled heart tones<br>→ Vascular: +2/4 bilaterally equal – ·radial ·femoral ·dorsalis pedis arteries<br>→ Abdomen: ·non tender (no guarding, |

| 59 | Should er Exam | .EDSH OULD ER | Left and Right Shoulder [Positive/Negative/Unknown – 38048]<br>· [Positive/Negative/Unknown] – drop arm test<br>· [Positive/Negative/Unknown] – empty can test<br>· [Positive/Negative/Unknown] – Yergason's test<br>· [Positive/Negative/Unknown] – Hawkins-Kennedy<br>· [Positive/Negative/Unknown] – Spurling's test<br>· [Positive/Negative/Unknown] – Adson's test |
| --- | --- | --- | --- |

| 60 | Trauma Exam | .TRAUMAEXAM | Primary Assessment → General: ·alert and oriented ·patient in cervical collar ·no distress noted<br>→ Airway and Breathing: ·airway patent ·spontanoues respirations ·ventilated ·vesicular breath sounds – clear bilaterally<br>→ Circulation: ·skin is warm ·well perfused<br>→ Disability: ·Glasgow Coma Scale – eye opening response, verbal response, motor response<br>→ Exposure: ·clothing was cut ·warm blankets applied ·severe burnt wound<br>Secondary Assessment → HEENT: · Head – ·normocephalic ·atraumatic<br>· Eyes – ·pupils equal, round and reactive<br>· Ears – ·otorrhea ·heamotympanum<br>· Nose – ·epitaxis ·septal hematoma<br>· Throat – ·oropharynx clear ·pink ·moist ·active bleeding or intraoral injuries<br>→ Neck: ·trachea midline ·no Jugular Venous DIstension ·no midline C spine tenderness<br>→ Chest: ·symmetrical chest movement ·non-tender chest wall ·no crepitus ·no subcutaneous emphysema ·lungs are clear on auscultations bilaterally<br>→ Cardiovascular: ·regular rate and rhythm of pulse ·normal S1 S2 sounds ·no murmurs ·no rubs ·no muffled heart tones<br>→ Vascular: +2/4 bilaterally equal – ·radial ·femoral ·dorsalis pedis arteries |

| 61 | Upper Extremity Strength Exam | UESTRENGTH | Strength 5/5 in: · Biceps<br>· Triceps<br>· Deltoids<br>· Wrist flexors and extensors<br>· Intrinsic muscles of hands |
| --- | --- | --- | --- |

# Emergency Department Course

| # | Terminology | Dot Phrase | Description |
| --- | --- | --- | --- |
| 62 | Labs | .THISVISITONLY | Auto-filling populates |
| 63 | Medications Administered | .MEDENCR | Auto-filling populates |
| 64 | Orders | .EDENCORDNM | Auto-filling populates |
| 65 | Radiology / Imaging | .EDWETREAD | → Imaging ordered and reviewed by Dr *** <br><br>→ Interpretated by radiology<br>→ Indication:<br>→ Interpretations Auto-filling populates |

# Procedures

| # | Terminology | Dot Phrase | Description |
|---|---|---|---|
| 66 | Arterial Blood Gas | .ABGPROC | → Procedure: arterial blood gas<br>→ Time: 00:00<br>→ Procedure performed by Dr ** of **radial arterial blood gas<br>→ No aesthetic was used<br>→ A total of **cc of blood was obtained<br>→ Direct pressure was held for *8 minutes<br>→ No complications, patient tolerated the procedure well |

| 67 | Arterial Line Placement | .EDARTERIALLINEPROC | → Procedure: arterial line placement<br>→ Time: 00:00<br>→ Procedure performed by Dr**<br>→ Procedure performed in sterile technique following standard protocol · Washing hands<br>· Cap, mask and sterile gown and gloves worn prior to procedure<br>→ Body area was cleansed using 2% chlorhexidine and was prepped and draped in a sterile manner<br>→ Arterial line placement was considered to (obtain multiple ABG/ avoid respiratory failure/ monitor hemodynamic stability)<br>→ Arterial line placed in (right/left) radial artery or (right/left) brachial artery or (right/left) femoral artery after area was anesthetized with **% of ** by Dr.**<br>→ Allen's test was normal/ not normal<br>→ A (18/20/22) gauge needle was used via **Seldinger technique and successful after **attempts<br>→ Post procedure – line was sutured/ dressing applied<br>→ Circulation, motor and sensory were (normal/unchanged/decreased circulation/weakness/numbness)<br>→ No immediate complications, patient tolerated the procedure well |

| 68 | Arterial Line Placement | .PARTERIALLINE | → Procedure: **arterial line placement<br>→ Time: 00:00<br>→ Indication: continuous blood pressure monitoring<br>→ Sterile technique was used and a **arterial line was placed<br>→ The body area was cleansed using **swabs, prepped and draped in a sterile manner<br>→ Artery canulated with introducer needle and guidewire was advanced through the introducer needle<br>→ Introducer needle was removed over guidewire and arterial catheter was slid into place without difficulties<br>→ Guidewire was removed and transducer line was connected showing a satisfactory waveform on monitor<br>→ Arterial catheter was secured and sutured using single 0 silk suture material<br>→ Patient tolerated procedure well |

| 69 | Arthroce ntesis | .ARTHRO CENTESI S | → Procedure: Arthrocentesis<br>→ Indication: rule out septic joint and/or acute gout<br>→ Procedure performed by Dr **<br>→ Consent obtained prior to procedure. All benefits, risks (including infection, bleeding, pain, nerve injury and hemarthrosis), complications, and alternative treatments discussed with patient. Questions, queries and concerns addressed<br>→ The ** joint was prepped and draped in sterile manner<br>→ Overlying skin and soft tissue was anesthetized with 2% lidocaine. Sterile 18G needle was used to aspirate fluid from joint which was sent to lab for evaluation and analysis<br>→ Approximately **mL aspirated<br>→ Patient's skin was cleansed with **and puncture site bandaged<br>→ Estimated blood loss **mL<br>→ No complications and patient tolerated the procedure |
|---|---|---|---|

| 70 | Cardiove rsion | .CARDIO VERSION | → Procedure: cardioversion<br>→ Time: 00:00<br>→ Procedure performed by Dr **<br>→ All benefits and risks of procedure were discussed to patient and caregiver/family<br>→ Written consent obtained by Dr**<br>→ Patient placed on telemetry, continuous pulse oximetry and **L NC oxygen<br>→ Peripheral IV line established<br>→ Medication/ no medication was given for successful sedation<br>→ **J biphasic synchronised shock provided ** amount of time resulting in restoration of ** rhythm with heart rate in **<br>→ EKG (as noted above)<br>→ No complications noted<br>→ Patients returned to normal mentation ** minutes following completion of procedure<br>→ No immediate complications, patient tolerated procedure well |
|---|---|---|---|

| 71 | Central Line Placement | .EDCENTRALLINEPROC | → Procedure: central line |
|---|---|---|---|
| | | | → Time: 00:00 |
| | | | → Indication: vascular access needed |
| | | | → Site was marked and ** was done using ultrasound guidance |
| | | | → Central line placement was performed with sterile technique · Washing hands |
| | | | · Cap, mask and sterile gown and gloves worn prior to procedure |
| | | | → The body area was cleansed using 2% chlorhexidine for cutaneous antiseptic, prepped and draped in a sterile manner |
| | | | → For anaesthesia **% of ** with **epinephrine and total of **mL was injected into site of interest |
| | | | → Central line placed by Dr ** |
| | | | → Access started in (right/left) subclavian/internal jugular/femoral |
| | | | → Patient positioned in ** |
| | | | → A (catheter size) of (catheter type – triple lumen catheter) was placed |
| | | | → Successful placement after **attempts |
| | | | → Adequate blood return was noted, and line was secured and sutured in place |
| | | | → No immediate complications, patient tolerated procedure well |

| 72 | Chest Tube Placement | .CHESTTUBE | → Procedure: chest tube placement<br>→ Time: 00:00<br>→ Procedure performed by: Dr **<br>→ Patient consent was obtained by Dr**<br>→ Left/ Right mid axillary line of chest wall of patient was prepped and draped following protocol sterile manner<br>→ Patient anesthetized with **% of ** of **cc<br>→ Incision with **blade made. Tissue bluntly dissected over superior part of rib penetrating thoracic cavity<br>→ Rush of air noted.<br>→ **chest tube passed into thoracic cavity. Tube secured and sutured in place with silk suture.<br>→ Site cleaned and occlusive dressing applied over chest tube<br>→ Chest tube position confirmed by Chest X ray<br>→ Expanded ** of left/ right lung noted<br>→ No immediate complications, patient tolerated procedure well |

| 73 | Conscious Sedation | .PROCSEDATION | → Procedure: procedural sedation<br>→ Time: 00:00<br>→ Aldrete score:<br>→ Time began:<br>→ Time ended:<br>→ Indication: anxiolysis and pain control to facilitate procedure<br>→ Time out – was performed<br>→ Pre-sedation checklist – reviewed and complete prior to sedation · Risk and benefits of moderate sedation discussed with patient and caregiver/family<br>· Risk of intubation discussed with patient and caregiver/family<br>· Patients last meal was greater than **hours prior to sedation<br>· Written consent obtained → Respiratory therapist and nursing staff is present at bedside for airway monitoring<br>→ Pre-procedural history and physical exam performed by ** prior to procedure<br>→ Patient placed on: · Cardiac monitory<br>· Pulse oximeter<br>· Supplement oxygen given via nasal cannula → Patient given ** of ** of **cc resulting in adequate sedation<br>→ Other procedure was completed, and patient was recovered from sedation according to protocol<br>→ I/myself was present in the room until patient's Aldrete score has returned 9<br>→ No complication during sedation |
| --- | --- | --- | --- |

| 74 | Consciou s Sedation | .ERSEDA TION | → Procedure: procedural sedation<br>→ Time: 00:00<br>→ Aldrete score:<br>→ Time began:<br>→ Time ended:<br>→ Indication: anxiolysis and pain control to facilitate procedure<br>→ Time out – was performed<br>→ Pre-sedation checklist – reviewed and complete prior to sedation<br>→ Diagnosis and system review:<br>→ Operation proposed:<br>→ Age (auto-filling populates)<br>→ Drug allergies (auto-filling populates)<br>→ Drug therapy (auto-filling populates)<br>→ Labs/blood sugar (auto-filling populated)<br>→ Anaesthetic history (auto-filling populated) · Risk and benefits of moderate sedation discussed with patient and caregiver/family<br>· Risk of intubation discussed with patient and caregiver/family<br>· Patients last meal was greater than **hours prior sedation<br>· Written consent obtained → Respiratory therapist and nursing staff is present at bedside for airway monitoring<br>→ Pre-procedural history and physical exam performed by ** prior to procedure<br>→ Patient placed on: · Cardiac monitory<br>· Pulse oximeter<br>· Supplement oxygen given via nasal cannula → Patient given ** |

| 75 | Digital Block | .DIGITAL BLOCK | → Procedure: digital block<br>→ Time: 00:00<br>→ Procedure performed by Dr **.<br>→ Consent obtained prior to procedure. All benefits, risks, complications, and alternative treatments discussed with patient. Questions, queries and concerns addressed<br>→ Base of **finger prepped in sterile fashion<br>→ Injection a total of **cc of 0.5% sensorcaine at base of (left or right) digital nerve<br>→ Block of successful<br>→ No complication<br>→ Patient tolerated procedure appropriately |
| 77 | EKG | .EDEKGI NTERPR ET | → Procedure: EKG. A 12 lead EKG was ordered, obtained and interpreted by Dr ***<br>→ Indication:<br>→ Interpretations: per my interpretation: · This showed - **<br>· Ventricular rate – beats per minutes<br>· PR interval – ms<br>· QRS duration – ms<br>· QTc interval – ms → Compared to an EKG dated ** and ** |

| 78 | Epistaxis Management | .EPISTAXISMANAGEMENT PROC | → Procedure: epistaxis management<br>→ Time: 00:00<br>→ Procedure performed by Dr **<br>→ Applied **% of ** anaesthesia to the right/left nostril and was left in place prior to procedure<br>→ Then **silver nitrate/ rhino rocket/ anterior pack was applied to the (right/left) anterior/posterior/ Kiesselbach's area<br>→ Post procedure bleeding stopped/ bleeding decreased/ no improved was noted<br>→ There was no recurrence of recent blood<br>→ No immediate complication, patient tolerated the procedure well |
| 79 | Fecal Disimpaction | .SHHFECALDISIMPACTION | → Procedure: fecal disimpaction<br>→ Using gloved finger with KY jelly manually disimpact (·small ·medium ·large – 100834) amount of hard feculent materials from rectum<br>→ Patient tolerated procedure well |

| 80 | Foreign Body Removal | .FOREIG BODYRE MOV | → Procedure: foreign body removal<br>→ Time: 00:00<br>→ Procedure performed by Dr **<br>→ Foreign body noted to body area/site<br>→ Body area anesthetized with **% of ** with or without epinephrine of total **cc used<br>→ Patient was/was not sedated and was/ was not restrained<br>→ Total of ** objects were recovered<br>→ ·all foreign bodies removed ·foreign body not removed ·residual foreign body remained<br>→ No immediate complication and patient tolerated procedure well |
| 81 | G-tube Placement | .GTUBE | → Patient presented with having feeding tube placed/**replaced<br>→ I gently dilated tube using **<br>→ A **gastronomy feeding tube was then advanced through the tract<br>→ Balloon cuff was inflated with **mL of sterile water<br>→ Post placement of KUB with contrast was ordered and reviewed showing feeding tube to be **<br>→ Patient tolerated the procedure well |

| 82 | G-tube Placement | .GTUBE | → Patient presented with having feeding tube placed/**replaced<br>→ I gently dilated tube using **<br>→ A **gastronomy feeding tube was then advanced through the tract<br>→ Balloon cuff was inflated with **mL of sterile water<br>→ Post placement of KUB with contrast was ordered and reviewed showing feeding tube to be **<br>→ Patient tolerated the procedure well |
| 83 | Imaging | .EDWET READ | → Imaging ordered and reviewed by Dr**<br>→ Interpretated by Radiology department<br>→ Indication:<br>→ Interpretation:<br>→ @wetread@ |

| 84 | Incision and Drainage | .INCISIONANDDRAINAGEPROC | → Procedure: incision and drainage<br>→ Time: 00:00<br>→ Procedure performed by Dr**<br>→ ·abscess ·cyst ·pilonidal cyst – seen on body site **<br>→ Area site was anesthetized with **% of ** with/without epinephrine. A total of **cc injected<br>→ A **blade scalpel was used making single straight incision to area<br>→ There was ·scant ·moderate ·copious amount of ·purulent ·serosangineous ·serous ·bloody drainage noted<br>→ No immediate complication and patient tolerated procedure appropriately |

| 85 | Intubation | .INTUBATION | → Procedure: intubation<br>→ Time: 00:00<br>→ Procedure performed by: Dr ** after indication of respiratory distress from patient.<br>→ Procedure completed via **direct oral/fibreoptic surgical/video ·patient was preoxygenated using (non-rebreather mask/ BVM) ·prior to intubation patient sedated using (** etomidate/fentanyl) ·Patient also given (succinylcholine/ vecurorium)<br>k·patient intubated using (**Miller/ Mac) with **tube size after **attempts ·after intubation positive colour change on $CO_2$ detector or chest rise with evidence of equal breath sound/absent breath sounds ·post intubation chest x-ray ordered ·interpretated by Dr** ·Interpretation showing ET tube in appropriate position /too high/too low → No immediate complication and patient tolerated procedure well |

| 86 | Intubation | .RSI | → Procedure: rapid sequence intubation<br>→ Time: 00:00<br>→ Patient pre-oxygenated with 100% O2.<br>→ Patient given **mg of ** then followed by **mg of **.<br>→ Patient intubated with **endotracheal tube; I visualised the tip of ED tube passing through vocal cords<br>→ Balloon cuff on ED tube was inflated<br>→ Patient was ventilated with Ambu bag<br>→ End tidal CO2 detector immediately changed from purple to yellow in colour<br>→ Presence of breath sounds auscultated over bilateral lung. Absence of air sounds on auscultation over epigastrium.<br>→ Tube secured by respiratory therapy<br>→ Using portable chest x-ray, it showed tip of ED to be **cm above carina and in satisfactory position<br>→ Patient tolerated procedure well |

| 87 | Joint Aspiration/ Arthrocentesis | .JOINTASPIRATION | → Procedure: Arthrocentesis<br>→ Indication: rule out septic joint and/or acute gout<br>→ Procedure performed by Dr **<br>→ Consent obtained prior to procedure. All benefits, risks (including infection, bleeding, pain, nerve injury and hemarthrosis), complications, and alternative treatments discussed with patient. Questions, queries and concerns addressed<br>→ The ** joint was prepped and draped in sterile manner<br>→ Overlying skin and soft tissue was anesthetized with **. Sterile 18G needle was used to aspirate fluid from joint which was sent to lab for evaluation and analysis<br>→ Approximately **mL aspirated<br>→ Patient's skin was cleansed of antiseptic and puncture site bandaged<br>→ No complications and patient tolerated the procedure |

| 88 | Joint Reduction | .JOINTREDUCTION | → Procedure: joint reduction |
| --- | --- | --- | --- |
| | | | → Indication: dislocated joint |
| | | | → Procedure performed by Dr ** |
| | | | → Consent obtained prior to procedure. All benefits, risks (including nerve injury and fracture), complications, and alternative treatments discussed with patient. Questions, queries and concerns addressed |
| | | | → A ** technique used |
| | | | → Joint was reduced on the ** attempt |
| | | | → Neurovascular status was rechecked and noted to be intact after procedure |
| | | | → Post reduction films ordered and revealed ** |
| | | | → No complications and patient tolerated the procedure |

| 89 | Laceratio n Repair | .EDLACE RATION | → Procedure: laceration repair<br>→ Laceration repair performed by: Dr**<br>→ Consent obtained prior to procedure. All benefits, risks, complications, and alternative treatments discussed with patient. Questions, queries and concerns addressed: ·a ** cm (size) laceration to the ** (site), anaesthetized using total of ** mL of ** locally.<br>→ Injection was performed by Dr **. Laceration site was cleaned and cleansed per nursing protocol. Laceration prepped in sterile fashion. Using sterile technique, the wound was initiated.<br>→ No evidence of any retained foreign body or injury to deep lying structures<br>→ Using ** (type of suture), a total of ** (number of sutures) were used to approximate the tissue edges<br>→ Patient tolerated procedure appropriately<br>→ Sterile dressing and triple ointment applied |
|---|---|---|---|

| 90 | Long Leg Posterior Mold Splint Application | .PLLPMS PLINT | → Procedure: long leg posterior mold splint placement<br>→ Using ** inch Ortho glass (type of splint) material, made and placed a ** long leg posterior mold splint<br>→ Splint ran from the tips of toes to the mid thigh, knee flexed to 30°C<br>→ Splint held in place using an Ace wrap<br>→ After splint placed, capillary refill <2seconds to all nail beds of the hand<br>→ Patients moves all ** - all pink, warm, and dry<br>→ Patient tolerated splint placement appropriately |

| 91 | Lumbar Puncture | .LUMBAR PUNCTURE | → Procedure: lumbar puncture<br>→ Time: 00:00<br>→ Patient consent was obtained by Dr**<br>→ Indication: to evaluate for infection or altered mental status or subarachnoid haemorrhage<br>→ Patient given **% of ** of **cc<br>→ Patient prepped and draped following protocol sterile manner<br>→ Patient position in sitting/ left lateral decubitus/ right lateral decubitus<br>→ Entered L3-L4 or L4-L5 interspace. 21-gauge 3in spinal needle used<br>→ ** attempts were made<br>→ Fluid appeared **. Total of ** tubes collected with total of ** mL volume<br>→ Site cleaned and pressure dressing applied with adhesive bandage<br>→ No immediate complications, patient tolerated procedure well |
| --- | --- | --- | --- |

| 92 | Lumbar Puncture | .PLUMBA RPUNCT URE | → Procedure: lumbar puncture<br>→ Time: 00:00<br>→ Patient consent was obtained by Dr**. Risks and benefits were discussed with patient and caregiver/ family · Risks included: procedure site, infection, bleeding, post dural headache → Indication: rule out SAH/ CNS infection<br>→ Patient position in left lateral decubitus with knees and hips and neck flexed<br>→ Patient prepped and draped following protocol sterile manner<br>→ Patient given **mL of **lidocaine anaesthetized L4-L5 interspace. Using **gauge spinal needle<br>→ ** attempts were made<br>→ Return of **CSF. A total of **mL of CSF collected in ** tubes<br>→ Site cleaned and pressure dressing applied with sterile band aid over puncture site<br>→ No immediate complications, patient tolerated procedure well<br>→ Patient can move all extremities<br>→ CSF sent to lab for microscopy and further analysis |
|---|---|---|---|

| 93 | Nail Avulsion | .NAILAVU LSION | → Procedure: nail avulsion<br>→ Digital block: patient was anesthetized **cc of ** in the **.<br>→ Nail was removed using sterile forceps and scissors<br>→ Wound cleansed using standard wound protocol with cida-stat. Additional cleaning saline irrigation and/or debridement ** performed<br>→ Wound explored: · No foreign bodies found<br>· No deep structure involvement<br>→ Some avulsions of nail bed and no body exposure<br>→ Wound prepped and draped in sterile manner<br>→ Patient nail was shaped using sterile scissors<br>→ Suture in place with ** 4-0 Vicryl sutures placed<br>→ Patient tolerated procedure well |
|---|---|---|---|
| 94 | Nail Trepanati on | .NLTREP H | → Procedure: nail trepanation<br>→ Time: 00:00<br>→ Procedure performed by Dr **<br>→ Patient's ** (which appendage) was anesthetized with digital block of 1% lidocaine of **mL<br>→ The ** was then trephinated with a heated cautery pen. One hole was burned through nail with release of the subungual hematoma<br>→ The ** was then soaked in Cida-Stat to facilitate further drainage of hematoma<br>→ No complications and patient tolerated the procedure |

| 95 | No Labs or Imaging performed by MDM | .HXPEX | Clinical history and physical examination do no warrant laboratory investigations and analysis or imaging at this time |
| 96 | NurseMaid Reduction | .NURSEMAIDREDUCTION | → Procedure: nursemaid's of upper extremity<br>→ Time: 00:00<br>→ Procedure performed by Dr **<br>→ Patient with history and physical exam suggesting or indicating nursemaid's elbow<br>→ Utilizing supination and flexion movement of the left/right elbow – palpable click was felt in flexion<br>→ CMS post procedure intact<br>→ With period of 5-10 minutes – the child is utilizing extremity normally<br>→ No complications and patient tolerated the procedure |

| 97 | Short Leg Posterior Mold Splint | .PSLPMS PLINT | → Procedure: short leg posterior mold splint placement<br>→ Using ** inch Ortho glass (type of splint) material, made and placed a ** short leg posterior mold splint<br>→ Splint ran from the tips of toes to the mid calf, ankle dorsiflexed to 90°C<br>→ Splint held in place using an Ace wrap<br>→ After splint placed, capillary refill <2seconds to all nail beds of the foot<br>→ Patients moves all ** - all pink, warm, and dry<br>→ Patient tolerated splint placement appropriately |

| 98 | Slit Lamp Exam – Foreign Body Removal | .SLITFOR EIGN | → Procedures: slit-lamp examination and foreign body removal<br>→ Time: 00:00<br>→ Patient consent was obtained by Dr**<br>→ Patient's left or right eye was examined with assistance from slit lamp and **proparacaine drops were administered<br>→ Foreign body was visualised at the **<br>→ Dr** and I were able/not able to remove foreign body with **<br>→ After removal, fluorescence uptake noted only to the abrasion left over from having remove foreign body<br>→ Patient eye irrigated with eyewash solution<br>→ Post-procedure, final slit lamp examination no indication of remaining foreign body<br>→ No immediate complications, patient tolerated procedure well |
| --- | --- | --- | --- |

| 99 | Slit Lamp Exam – General | .PSLITLAMPEXAM | ·slit-lamp exam was completes of patient's left/right eye ·there is ** matting or collerette formation involving eyelashes ·there is **periorbital edema or ecchymosis ·eye was examined through full range of motion ·**evidence of retained foreig body<br>·superior palpebra everted for evidence of foriegn body ·there is presence or absence of **hhyphema or **hypopyon<br>·anterior chambers are adequate and equal depth hbilaterally ·there is **cell or flare reaction ·evidence of corneal foriegn body → Eye was then stained with fluorescein strip and examined under cobalt light<br>→ Examination showed **<br>→ Patient tolerated the procedure well<br>→ **drops of proparacaine administered in eye ti provide relief of discomfort |
| 100 | Splint Application | .SPLINTAPPLICATION | → Procedure: splint application<br>→ Time: 00:00<br>→ Ortho glass (type of splint) was applied to the location by Dr **<br>→ Splinted body pare was neurovascularly intact following procedure<br>→ No immediate complication and patient tolerated procedure appropriately |

| 101 | Splint Application | .EDPROCEDURESPLINT | → Procedure: splint placement<br>→ Using ** inch Ortho glass (type of splint) material, made and placed a ** mold splint that ran from **to the**<br>→ Splint held in place using an Ace wrap<br>→ Patient tolerated splint placement appropriately<br>→ After splint placed, capillary refill <2seconds to all nail beds of the **<br>→ Patients moves all ** - all pink, warm, and dry |
| --- | --- | --- | --- |
| 102 | Thumb Spica Splint | .TSSPLINT | → Procedure: thumb spica splint placement<br>→ Using ** inch Ortho glass (type of splint) material, made and placed a ** thumb spica splint<br>→ Splint ran from the thumb to mid forearm, wrist dorsiflexed to 15°C<br>→ Splint held in place using an Ace wrap<br>→ After splint placed, capillary refill <2seconds to all nail beds of the hand<br>→ Patients moves thumb - had good sensation to the thumb - all pink, warm, and dry<br>→ Patient tolerated splint placement appropriately |

| 103 | Ulnar Gutter Splint | .UGSPLINT | → Procedure: ulnar gutter splint placement<br>→ Using ** inch Ortho glass (type of splint) material, made and placed a ** ulnar gutter splint<br>→ Splint ran from the ** to mid forearm, wrist dorsiflexed to 15°C<br>→ Splint held in place using an Ace wrap<br>→ After splint placed, capillary refill <2seconds to all nail beds of the hand<br>→ Patients moves all ** - had good sensation to the fingertips - all pink, warm, and dry<br>→ Patient tolerated splint placement appropriately |
| --- | --- | --- | --- |

# Calls – Consults – Recheck

| # | Terminology | Dot Phrase | Description |
| --- | --- | --- | --- |
| 104 | Pelvic Exam Performed | .GUEXAM | → Time: 00:00<br>→ Pelvic exam was performed with female ER staff member present in examination room<br>→ Findings: |
| 105 | Physician calls | .CALL | → Time: 00:00<br>→ Discussed patient's case with Dr ** (**) |
| 106 | Quick Discharge After Initial Evaluation | .QUICK/ EDQUICK DISCHARGE | → Time: 00:00<br>→ Finished ** and discussed plan for discharge and follow up with the patient (name)<br>→ Patient ** was in agreement with the discussed plan<br>→ All questions and queries were answered<br>→ **return to ED instructions were also discussed presently |

| 107 | Recheck with RN | .HUDDLE | → Time: 00:00<br>→ Admission/ discharge ** huddle completed with nurse **<br>→ All diagnostic laboratory investigations and images were reviewed, discussed for a management, treatment and follow up plan<br>→ Patient (name) understands and was in agreement |
| --- | --- | --- | --- |
| 108 | Recheck/Re-evaluation | .RECHECK | → Time: 00:00<br>→ Rechecked patient who is resting comfortably<br>→ Laboratory investigations ** and imaging ** results were discussed<br>→ Discussed plans for discharge and follow up with the patient (name)<br>→ Patient ** was in agreement with the discussed plan<br>→ All questions and queries were answered |
| 109 | Wisconsin Prescription Drug Monitoring Program Check | .WIRX/.WISPDMP | → Reviewed the Wisconsin Prescription Drug Monitoring Program Website<br>→ Found: |

# Medical Decision Making

| # | Terminology | Dot Phrase | Description |
| --- | --- | --- | --- |

| 110 | General: Medical Decision Making | .EDM DM | → The patient is a (age) (sex) who presents to the ed with chief complaint of **<br>→ EPIC records were reviewed<br>→ Laboratory investigations were ordered and reviewed<br>→ Findings stated above<br>→ A diagnostic ** was additionally ordered and reviewed<br>→ Imaging interpretation shows **<br>→ EKG was performed and revealed a **<br>→ Cardiac monitoring and oximeter were placed during the patient's ED stay<br>→ Patient provided with *** resulting in ** of symptoms alleviation<br>→ Patient was discharged with a diagnosis of ***<br>→ Patient advised to **; recommended for the patient to follow up with **<br>→ The patient provided with prescriptions for **<br>→ Patient's vital signs and condition *** during evaluation in the ED<br>→ Patient (name) was in agreement with plan of care<br>→ All questions, queries and concerns were addressed appropriately |

| 111 | Medical Decision Making | .EDM<br>DM | → The patient is a (age) (sex) who presented to the ED with a chief complaint of ***<br>→ EPIC records were reviewed<br>→ Patient was placed on cardiac monitor and oximeter<br>→ Multiple differential diagnosis evaluated including ***.<br>→ IV line was inserted<br>→ Laboratory investigations and imaging was ordered and reviewed<br>→ Findings stated above<br>→ EKG was obtained showing ***<br>→ The patient provided with *** resulting in *** of symptoms alleviation.<br>→ Findings and warning symptomology were discussed with the patient (name)<br>→ The patient's vital signs and condition *** during evaluation in the ED<br>→ All questions and concerns were addressed. |

| 112 | Medical Decision Making | .EDM DM | → The patient is a (age) (sex) who presented to the ED with a chief complaint of ***<br>→ Initial vital signs and EPIC records were reviewed<br>→ Upon arrival patient (name) appeared **<br>→ Physical examination was significant ** as positives signs and ** as negative signs<br>→ Evaluation of ** with indicated for **<br>→ Patient provided with (medication/ IV fluids) resulting in *** of symptoms alleviation.<br>→ The routine and diagnostic work up of patient was significant for ** and presently will ** require admission<br>→ The patient's vital signs and condition *** during evaluation in the ED<br>→ All questions and concerns were addressed. |

| 113 | Medical Decision Making | .EDM DM | → The patient is a (age) (sex) who presented to the ED with a chief complaint of *** |

→ The patient is a (age) (sex) who presented to the ED with a chief complaint of ***

→ Vitals and physical examination are significant for **

→ EPIC records were reviewed

→ Differential diagnosis considered include **

→ Laboratory investigations and imaging was ordered and reviewed

→ Findings stated above

→ Additionally, a ** was ordered and reviewed showing ***

→ EKG was performed revealing **

→ Cardiac monitoring and oximeter were placed during the patient's ED stay

→ The patient provided with *** resulting in *** of symptoms alleviation

→ Patient was discharged with a diagnosis of **

→ It was recommended for the patient to call ** to schedule a follow up appointment and return to the **ED if symptoms worsen

→ Patient provided prescriptions for **

→ The patient's vital signs and condition *** were closely observed during evaluation in the ED

→ Patient was in agreement with the plan for care

→ All questions and concerns were addressed.

| 114 | Medical Decision Making | .EDM DM | → The patient is a (age) (sex) who presented to the ED with a chief complaint of ***<br>→ EPIC records were reviewed<br>→ Multiple diagnosis considered<br>→ Laboratory investigations and imaging was ordered and reviewed<br>→ Findings stated above<br>→ Additionally, a ** was ordered and reviewed<br>→ Imaging shows **<br>→ EKG was performed revealing **<br>→ Cardiac monitoring and oximeter were placed during the patient's ED stay<br>→ The patient provided with *** for symptoms<br>→ Patient was discharged with a diagnosis of **<br>→ Patient was advised to ** and further recommended to follow up with ** (specialist)<br>→ Patient provided prescriptions for **<br>→ The patient's vital signs and condition *** were closely observed during evaluation in the ED<br>→ Patient was in agreement with the plan for care<br>→ All questions and concerns were addressed<br>→ Patient care was supervised by Dr **<br>→ Physician to co-sign the note |

# Medical Decision Making Add-Ons

| # | Terminology | Dot Phrase | Description |
| --- | --- | --- | --- |
| 115 | Critical Care Time | .TDCRITCARE | → Critical care time: **minutes<br>→ Critical care time entailed:<br>· Direct bedside evaluation<br>· Formulating and directing treatment plans<br>· Speaking with consultants<br>· Excluding evaluation of other patients<br>· Excluding outside any billable procedures |
| 116 | Critical Care Time | .CRITCARE | → Critical care time in:<br>→ Critical care time out:<br>→ Total critical care time:<br>→ Critical care time entailed:<br>· Direct bedside evaluation<br>· Formulating and directing treatment plans<br>· Speaking with consultants<br>· Excluding evaluation of other patients<br>· Excluding outside any billable procedures |
| 117 | No Labs or Imaging Obtained | .HXPEX | Clinical history and physical examination do no warrant laboratory investigations and analysis or imaging at this time |

| 118 | Pneumonia Quality Indicator | .PNEUMONIAQUALITYINDICATOR | Quality Indication: pneumonia<br>1.　Patient's current mental status is stable - **<br>2.　Pulse oximetry on room air is - **%<br>3.　Empiric antibiotics - ** initiated Auto filling populates |

# Final Impression

| # | Terminology | Dot Phrase | Description |
| --- | --- | --- | --- |
| 119 | Diagnosis | .DXS | Auto filling populates |

# Plan

| # | Terminology | Dot Phrase | Description |
| --- | --- | --- | --- |
| 120 | Admit | .ADMIT | → Patient was admitted to hospital in stable condition<br>→ Patient was under the care of Dr ** for further evaluation and treatment |
| 121 | Discharge | .EDDC | → Patient discharged in ** condition<br>→ All questions and concerns were discussed, and no further questions or concerns were raised<br>→ Discharge instructions attachments included ** |
| 122 | Discharge Instruction | .EDDISCHARGEINSTRUCTIONS | Auto filling populates |
| 123 | Disposition | .EDDISPO | Auto filling populates |

| 124 | Prescription | .EDRXMEDSTART | Auto filling populates |

# Miscellaneous

| # | Terminology | Dot Phrase | Description |
| --- | --- | --- | --- |

| 125 | Blood Pressure Elevated with no diagnosis of hypertension (place in discharge instructions) | .EDBP | → During ED stay blood pressure was found to be higher than average<br>→ High blood pressure is not commonly diagnosed in ED due to multiple other factors that significantly contribute to the reading<br>→ Elevated blood pressure reading may be due to undiagnosed high blood pressure<br>→ It would be recommended that a recheck of the blood pressure is performed<br>→ Please call to schedule a recheck at your earliest convenience |

| 126 | Scribe disclaimer | .SCRIBEDISC LAIMER | → I, **, am serving as a scribe to document services personally performed by (HCP name**) based on my observation and HCP's statements directed towards me |
| 127 | Shift change | .SCRIBESHIF TCHANGE | → Time: 00:00<br>→ I, **, am assuming scribe role for this document for time noted above for (name)** |

| 128 | Use when the patient received a CT scan with IV contrast and is on Metformin (placed in discharge instructions) | .EDMETFORMIN | → You have been injected contrast dye and you are a known patient taking metformin<br>→ It would be recommended to HOLD your metformin medication for at least 48 hours<br>→ Contact your doctor within that period of withhold for a re-evaluation |

# COVID-19 Particulars

| # | Terminology | Dot Phrase | Description |
| --- | --- | --- | --- |
| 129 | Additional Medical Problems with COVID-19 | .ADDITIONAL MEDPROBLEMS | → Patients with such co-morbidities are at a higher risk of obtaining COVID-19 infection · Heart related diseases · Diabetes mellitus · Respiratory diseases · Dementia |

| 130 | Clinical presentation of COVID-19 in older patients | .COVID19OLDERPATIENTS | → Most common symptoms include: · Fever · Cough · Shortness of breath → Uncommon symptoms include: · Malaise · Confusion → Severe symptoms include: · Shortness of breath · Pain or pressure in chest · New confusion or somnolence · Bluish lips and face |

## Conclusions

The above dot phrases are some of our examples, feel free to use the available examples and build on them in your medical practice.

We hope you will use this book to save time and be more efficient and accurate in your medical practice.

**Please remember to leave a review online and help others find this book!**